ONE DAY AT A TIME

2018 DIARY

A Year-Long Journey of Personal Healing
and Transformation

Abby Wynne

GILL BOOKS

Gill Books

Hume Avenue

Park West

Dublin 12

www.gillbooks.ie

Gill Books is an imprint of M.H. Gill and Co.

© Abby Wynne 2017

978 07171 7957 2

Designed by Jane Matthews

For permission to reproduce photographs, the author and

publisher gratefully acknowledge the following:

© iStock: 2, 5, 11, 13, 14, 26, 36, 38, 50, 62, 75, 86, 98, 110, 122, 135, 146.

Printed by BZ Graf, Poland.

This book is typeset in Neutraface.

The paper used in this book comes from the wood pulp of managed forests.

For every tree felled, at least one tree is planted, thereby renewing natural resources.

A CIP catalogue record for this book is available from the British Library.

5 4 3 2

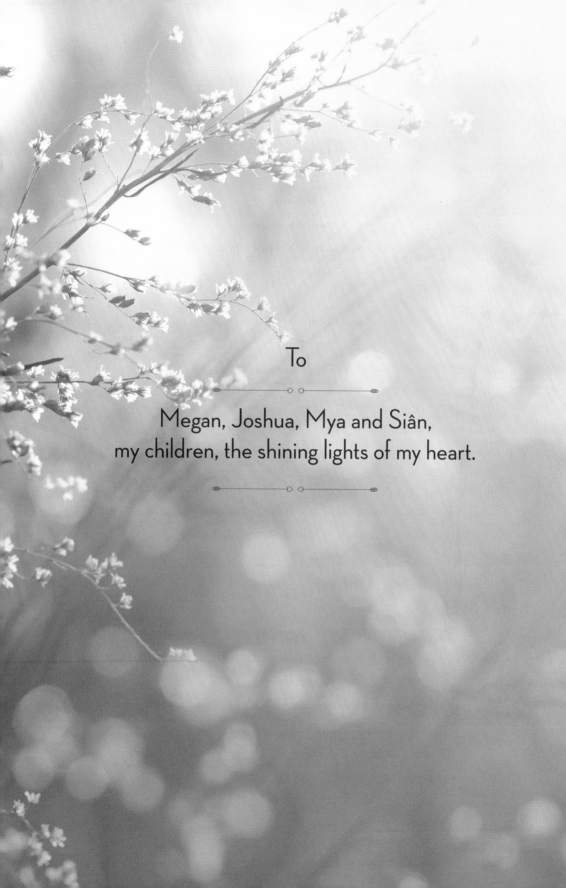

To

Megan, Joshua, Mya and Siân,
my children, the shining lights of my heart.

ABOUT THE AUTHOR

Abby Wynne is a shamanic psychotherapist, energy healer and published author based in Ireland. Abby teaches people how to connect their mind, heart and soul to access their inner wisdom, let go of fear and become more available for life.

Abby has recorded many guided meditations and healing sessions, all available on her website. Her previous books include *A–Z Spiritual Colouring Affirmations*, *How to Be Well* and *Energy Healing for Everyone*. She also runs regular online classes and group healing sessions. She sees clients in her private practice in Dublin or via Skype.

You can follow Abby on Facebook 'Abby's Energy Healing Page', Instagram @abbynrghealing, Twitter @abbynrghealing or sign up on www.abby-wynne.com to receive weekly energy tips by email.

Abby has recorded a copy of all of the affirmations in this book onto an audio file, and has also recorded copies of the exercises and visualisations to help you go deeper. These are available for free via www.abby-wynne.com/onedayatatime.

'Perhaps the most "spiritual" thing any of us can do is simply to look through our own eyes, see with eyes of wholeness, and act with integrity and kindness.'

Jon Kabat-Zinn

Name ....

Address ....

Telephone ....

Emergency contact ....

USEFUL DATES
2018

January 2018
Monday 1 .... New Year's Day

February 2018
Wednesday 14 .... Valentine's Day, Ash Wednesday (Lent begins)

March 2018
Sunday 11 .... Mother's Day
Saturday 17 .... St Patrick's Day
Monday 19 .... St Patrick's Day Bank Holiday
Sunday 25 .... Palm Sunday
Friday 30 .... Good Friday

April 2018
Sunday 1 .... Easter Sunday
Monday 2 .... Easter Monday

May 2018
Monday 7 .... May Day Bank Holiday

June 2018
Monday 4 .... June Bank Holiday
Sunday 17 .... Father's Day

August 2018
Monday 6 .... August Bank Holiday

October 2018
Monday 29 .... October Bank Holiday

December 2018
Monday 24 .... Christmas Eve
Tuesday 25 .... Christmas Day
Wednesday 26 .... St Stephen's Day
Monday 31 .... New Year's Eve

MOON PHASES CALENDAR
2018

January	2 ○	8 ◐	17 ●	24 ◑	31 ○
February	7 ◐	15 ●	23 ◑		
March	2 ○	9 ◐	17 ●	24 ◑	31 ○
April	8 ◐	16 ●	22 ◑	30 ○	
May	8 ◐	15 ●	22 ◑	29 ○	
June	6 ◐	13 ●	20 ◑	28 ○	
July	6 ◐	13 ●	19 ◑	27 ○	
August	4 ◐	11 ●	18 ◑	26 ○	
September	3 ◐	9 ●	17 ◑	25 ○	
October	2 ◐	9 ●	16 ◑	24 ○	31 ◐
November	7 ●	15 ◑	23 ○	30 ◐	
December	7 ●	15 ◑	22 ○	29 ◐	

SPECIAL MOON EVENTS
2018

Tuesday 2 January	Super Full Moon
Wednesday 17 January	Micro New Moon
Wednesday 31 January	Blue Moon (second full moon in single calendar month)
February	Black Moon (no Full Moon in calendar month)
Sunday 31 March	Blue Moon (second full moon in single calendar month)*
Friday 13 July	Super Full Moon
Friday 27 July	Micro Full Moon
Friday 27 to Saturday 28 July	Total Lunar Eclipse
Sunday 11 August	Super New Moon

*Two blue moons in a year is a rare event (second Full Moon in single calendar month)

CALENDAR
2018

JANUARY
Mo	Tu	We	Th	Fr	Sa	Su
1	2	3	4	5	6	7
8	9	10	11	12	13	14
15	16	17	18	19	20	21
22	23	24	25	26	27	28
29	30	31				

FEBRUARY
Mo	Tu	We	Th	Fr	Sa	Su
			1	2	3	4
5	6	7	8	9	10	11
12	13	14	15	16	17	18
19	20	21	22	23	24	25
26	27	28				

MARCH
Mo	Tu	We	Th	Fr	Sa	Su
			1	2	3	4
5	6	7	8	9	10	11
12	13	14	15	16	17	18
19	20	21	22	23	24	25
26	27	28	29	30	31	

APRIL
Mo	Tu	We	Th	Fr	Sa	Su
						1
2	3	4	5	6	7	8
9	10	11	12	13	14	15
16	17	18	19	20	21	22
23	24	25	26	27	28	29
30						

MAY
Mo	Tu	We	Th	Fr	Sa	Su
	1	2	3	4	5	6
7	8	9	10	11	12	13
14	15	16	17	18	19	20
21	22	23	24	25	26	27
28	29	30	31			

JUNE
Mo	Tu	We	Th	Fr	Sa	Su
				1	2	3
4	5	6	7	8	9	10
11	12	13	14	15	16	17
18	19	20	21	22	23	24
25	26	27	28	29	30	

JULY
Mo	Tu	We	Th	Fr	Sa	Su
						1
2	3	4	5	6	7	8
9	10	11	12	13	14	15
16	17	18	19	20	21	22
23	24	25	26	27	28	29
30	31					

AUGUST
Mo	Tu	We	Th	Fr	Sa	Su
		1	2	3	4	5
6	7	8	9	10	11	12
13	14	15	16	17	18	19
20	21	22	23	24	25	26
27	28	29	30	31		

SEPTEMBER
Mo	Tu	We	Th	Fr	Sa	Su
					1	2
3	4	5	6	7	8	9
10	11	12	13	14	15	16
17	18	19	20	21	22	23
24	25	26	27	28	29	30

OCTOBER
Mo	Tu	We	Th	Fr	Sa	Su
1	2	3	4	5	6	7
8	9	10	11	12	13	14
15	16	17	18	19	20	21
22	23	24	25	26	27	28
29	30	31				

NOVEMBER
Mo	Tu	We	Th	Fr	Sa	Su
			1	2	3	4
5	6	7	8	9	10	11
12	13	14	15	16	17	18
19	20	21	22	23	24	25
26	27	28	29	30		

DECEMBER
Mo	Tu	We	Th	Fr	Sa	Su
					1	2
3	4	5	6	7	8	9
10	11	12	13	14	15	16
17	18	19	20	21	22	23
24	25	26	27	28	29	30
31						

HOW TO USE THIS DIARY

There are several ways to use this diary, and however you choose to use it is up to you. You may drift between going deep and going light, depending on how you are feeling – a year is a long time, though it can pass very quickly. Whatever you choose to do, think of this diary as a guide who brings you to places you may never have imagined going to on your own, and as a friend, who gently reminds you to treat yourself better. I have written everything in the present tense to bring you into the present moment. Read as if you are saying the words to yourself, as there is great power in that.

You can of course simply enjoy the flow of the graphics and phrases, using the spaces provided to write down your appointments, just as you would with any other diary. To go deeper, you can pay attention to the affirmations and visualisations as they appear, and try the exercises. Each affirmation, exercise and visualisation is designed to be more effective the more you try it. In this way, you can start a year-long journey of personal healing and transformation.

THEMES

Every month has a theme. Schedule some time at the beginning of each month to sit and think about the monthly themes and intentions. Read them out loud, change or adjust them if you wish, then claim them as your own. One month you may delve deep into the theme, another month you may not. That's perfectly fine. Some of the monthly themes may call on you to dive in more than others.

AFFIRMATIONS

Different phrases accompany every week. Say the affirmations out loud a few times and with great feeling, knowing that each word has a vibration. Let the energy of the words pour inside you and allow their richness to guide you back to your heart when you become too entangled in life's difficulties. You can use the affirmations as a remedy or a treatment for any emotional upset you are feeling. Use them to help clear or change something in you. The more you say the affirmations and truly believe them, the more heaviness and emotional pain will be released. Try them all, even the ones you don't love so much, until you feel a difference inside.

EXERCISES

The exercises will help you relax and be more present. Attempt them more than once if necessary. Underline your favourites and come back to them until you break free from what is blocking you and break through to joy. Let compassion flow into your life, into every moment. Know that you're making the world a better place by making your energy brighter and stronger.

PROMPTS

At the beginning of each month, I have included some prompts to help you get started with your daily writing. Choose one for each day of the week, or make up your own.

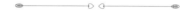

Let all of the elements of this diary – the graphics, affirmations and exercises – guide you inwards. On any page, feel free to write and scribble what comes up for you; this is your book. Buy yourself an additional notebook if you have more writing to do. If you really feel resistant to any of the themes, affirmations or exercises, perhaps those are the ones you need to work with! Don't be afraid to ask for help if doing some of the work here brings up emotional issues for you. Nothing beats a cuppa and a chat with a trusted friend. I have made joy and love the focus of the work for this year, but sometimes removing the internal blocks to these emotions can hurt.

All I ask of you is that you accept yourself, wherever you are right now on your journey. When you accept yourself and allow yourself to truly become who you are, contentment, peace and happiness naturally flow in. Don't punish yourself with expectations that you need to become a better person, because you don't. You may just need to be nicer to yourself, learn to accept yourself more and to become more aware of the choices you are making in your life and how they impact you.

So please – no pushing, no pressure, no expectations. Choose acceptance, love and compassion. Listen to your inner wisdom; you know what is best for you. Trust yourself.

And take it one day at a time.

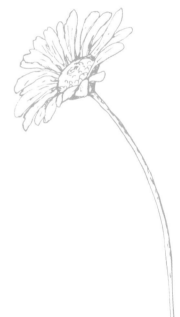

POWER STATEMENT

A power statement sets out your intentions for the coming year.
You can write your own power statement or use the one that I offer
you here. Come back to read your power statement often to remind
yourself of your direction and your intention for 2018. If you want to,
you can make a commitment to shift something heavy in you this year,
so that at the end of the year you feel lighter in yourself, happier
about your life, and that you have let in more love.

My Power Statement for 2018

'This year I want to look after myself
better. This year I commit to learning
who I am and what I like. I commit to
enjoying life without guilt, expressing
my creativity without fear and living a
life filled with purpose, love, joy and
inspiration.'

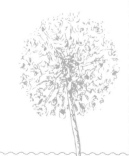

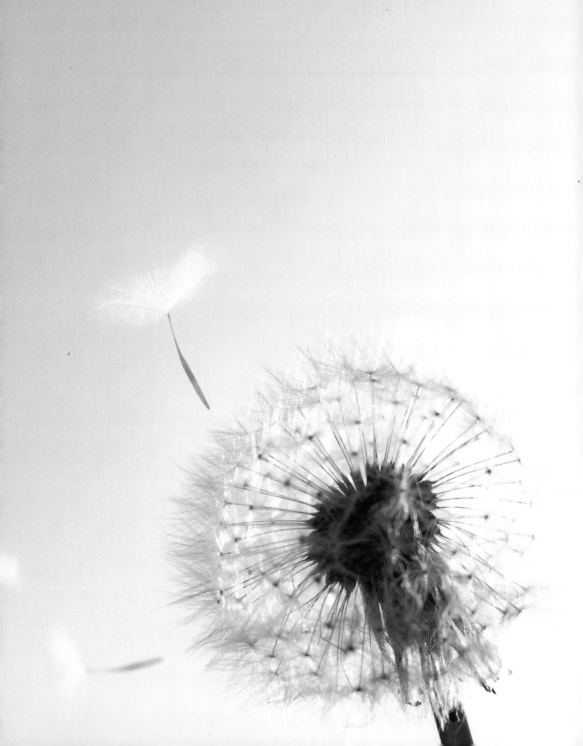

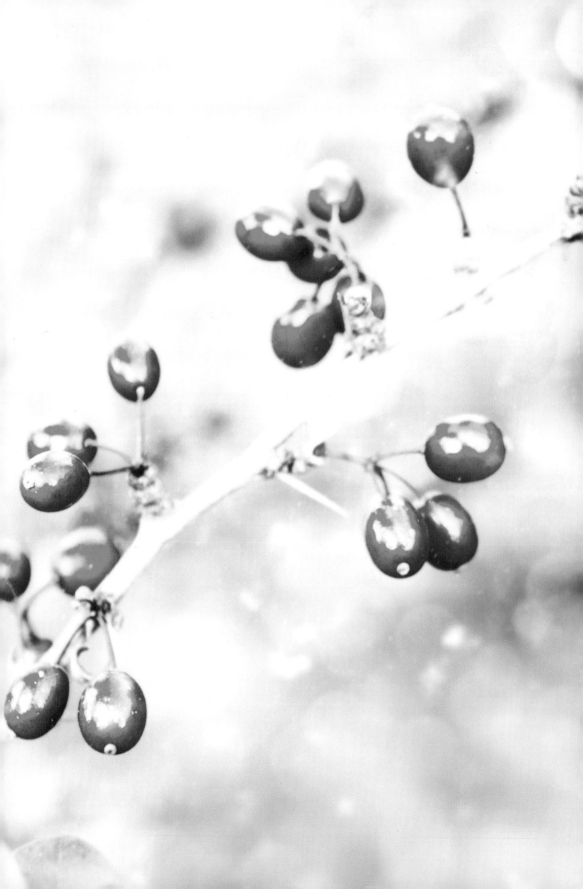

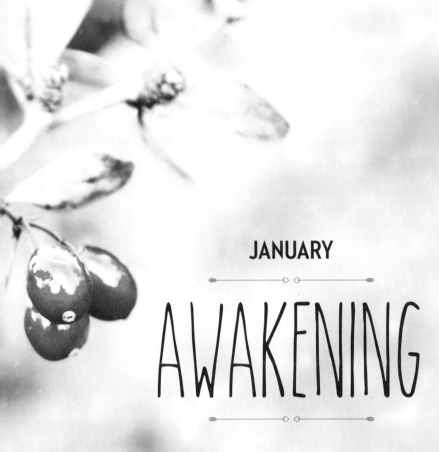

JANUARY

AWAKENING

This month I become the observer of my life.

'Your vision will become clear only when you can
look into your own heart. Who looks outside, dreams;
who looks inside, awakes.'

Carl Jung

JANUARY

I allow myself to gently awaken to the truth of how I have been treating myself. I know I need to invest in and nurture my relationship with myself. I am learning not to be afraid of change. I take the risk to grow so that I can create a better life for myself, become more aware of my choices and take one small step at a time. I am willing to take this first step and I am certain that my other relationships will naturally improve. With compassion I will take note of how I speak to myself and start to be nicer to myself. I know that it is worthwhile to take the necessary time to repair and heal. I can gently move towards kindness and treat myself with the love with which I want to treat others. When I have a good relationship with myself, I have a good relationship with the world.

Don't forget to use your prompts:
Today I will... Today I am... Today I think...
Today I feel... Today I believe... Today I trust... Today I can ...

EXERCISE:
When I catch myself speaking in a negative way towards myself, I write down the exact words that I used. In this way I can become more familiar with them. I will recognise the harsh words the next time and then deliberately choose compassionate words instead. So when I catch myself slipping into negativity, I say, 'I no longer need to hurt myself this way, I am doing the best that I can', and then I say my new words instead. Soon I find that my compassionate words replace the hurtful words and I feel more at peace with myself.

MONDAY 1

I step out of the way so I can see things as they really are.

TUESDAY 2

WEDNESDAY 3

I give myself permission to become aware of my thoughts.

THURSDAY 4

FRIDAY 5

I am still learning; I forgive myself and I move on.

SATURDAY 6

SUNDAY 7

I feel safe to grow and heal.

MONDAY 8

I have all the time that I need to make the changes that I want to make.

TUESDAY 9

WEDNESDAY 10

I am kind and gentle to myself.

THURSDAY 11

FRIDAY 12

I forgive myself for the mistakes that I have made.

SATURDAY 13

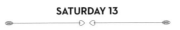

SUNDAY 14

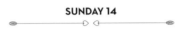

I allow myself to let go of anger and emotional pain.

MONDAY 15

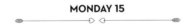

I feel strengthened and encouraged by the possibilities for my life.

TUESDAY 16

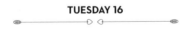

WEDNESDAY 17

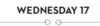

I catch myself and gently correct myself if needed.

THURSDAY 18

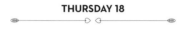

I give myself permission to let go of what I no longer need.

FRIDAY 19

I choose to have more love, beauty and joy in my life.

SATURDAY 20

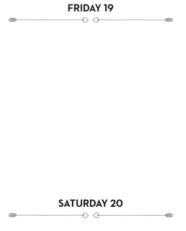

SUNDAY 21

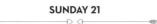

I let go of fearful thoughts and choose love instead.

MONDAY 22

I choose not to take things personally.

TUESDAY 23

WEDNESDAY 24

Everyone is doing the best that they can with what they know.

THURSDAY 25

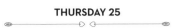

I am learning how to make better choices.

FRIDAY 26

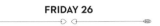

SATURDAY 27

I let go of my need to control things and to always be right.

SUNDAY 28

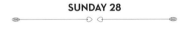

I am kind to myself as I learn how to look after myself.

MONDAY 29

I have compassion and kindness towards myself.

TUESDAY 30

WEDNESDAY 31

I am learning how to give myself what I need.

NOTES ON AWAKENING

January

WHAT DID I LEARN ABOUT MYSELF THIS MONTH?

HOW CAN I BE MORE COMPASSIONATE TOWARDS MYSELF NEXT MONTH?

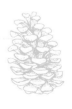

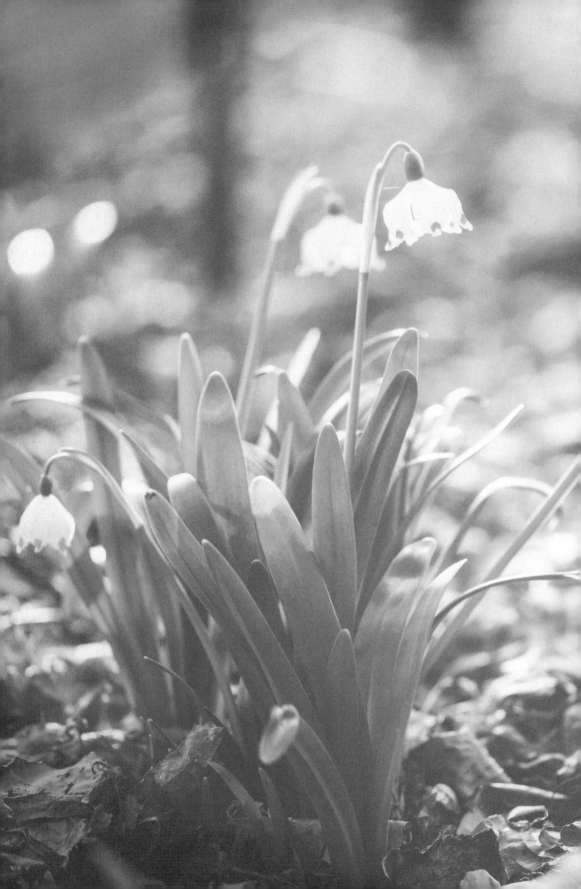

FEBRUARY

PRESENCE

This month I feel more at ease with myself.

'If your mind carries a heavy burden of past, you will experience more
of the same. The past perpetuates itself through lack of presence.
The quality of your consciousness at this moment is
what shapes the future.'

Eckhart Tolle

FEBRUARY

As compassion now flows from within me, I realise that it is safe to be more present in my life. I can bring myself more and more into the moment and connect with what is right in front of me instead of living in the past or in the future. I see what is actually in front of me instead of what I think is in front of me. I will discover that things I thought were difficult become easier when I am more present. I will realise that worrying does not enhance my life and that I prefer to be at peace. Choosing peace in every moment heals my body, mind and soul.

Don't forget to use your prompts:
Today I will... Today I am... Today I think...
Today I feel... Today I believe... Today I trust... Today I can ...

EXERCISE:
I feel my feet on the ground. I feel connection to this earth. I am here. I slow down my breath and bring my awareness and my presence into my body: into my feet (breath), my knees (breath), my hips (breath), my stomach (breath), my heart (breath), my shoulders (breath), my chest (breath), my face (breath), the top of my head (breath). I can hear my breath. I am safe. I am here.

THURSDAY 1
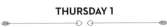

I feel my feet on the ground and I know that I am safe.

FRIDAY 2
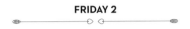

SATURDAY 3
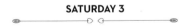

I bring myself into the present moment.

SUNDAY 4

PRESENCE

MONDAY 5

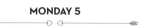

I let go of my need to control situations outside of myself.

TUESDAY 6

I feel safe to let go of my worries.

WEDNESDAY 7

THURSDAY 8

I am learning how to be my own best friend.

FRIDAY 9

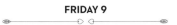

SATURDAY 10

I allow myself to have a life that I love.

SUNDAY 11

I choose to let go of all grudges and anger.

MONDAY 12

I connect to my heart and kindness flows into everything I say and do.

TUESDAY 13

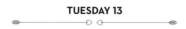

I step away from my thoughts and take time to see what is in front of me.

WEDNESDAY 14

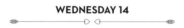

I am the centre of my universe.

THURSDAY 15

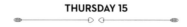

FRIDAY 16

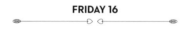

I choose to fill my world with peace and love.

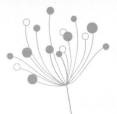

SATURDAY 17

SUNDAY 18

I don't need to carry the pain of the past into the present moment.

MONDAY 19

I slow down and pull my awareness into myself.

TUESDAY 20

I give myself complete permission to relax.

WEDNESDAY 21

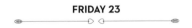

THURSDAY 22

I let go of my need to control; I realise I never controlled anything anyway.

FRIDAY 23

It is safe to be here. It is safe to let love in.

SATURDAY 24

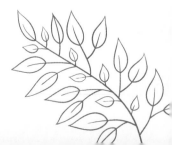

SUNDAY 25

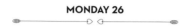

I accept myself for who I am and I accept others for who they are.

MONDAY 26

I connect to my intuition and listen to my inner wisdom.

TUESDAY 27

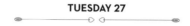

I unhook myself from the past and the future.

WEDNESDAY 28

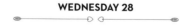

I can fully enjoy all that is here in this moment.

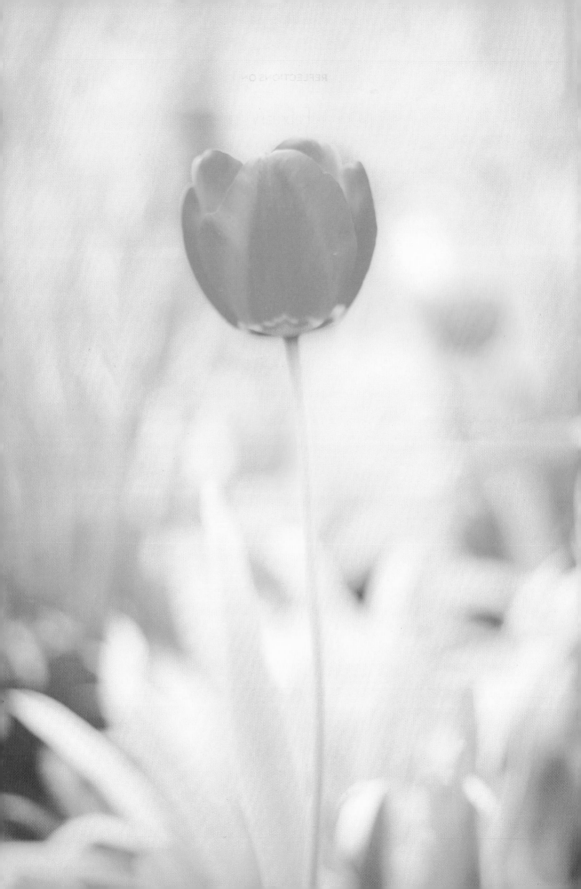

February

WHAT BROUGHT ME THE MOST PEACE THIS MONTH AND WHY?

WHAT WOULD I LIKE TO CONTINUE WORKING ON NEXT MONTH?

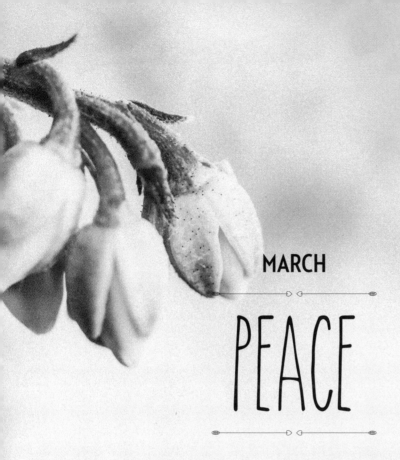

MARCH

PEACE

**This month I will continue the work
of improving my relationship with myself.**

'When you have peace within,
real peace with others is possible.'

Thich Nhat Hanh

MARCH

I will notice that it gets easier to be nice to myself, even in my thoughts. I will feel kindness reflected back to me in my life. I will notice that I have more energy and that I really enjoy the simple things in life. I know there is more work to do, but I am no longer afraid of it. I slowly release any resentment, anger and grudges that I've been harbouring against myself and others. As nature awakens after winter and growth begins, I too feel as if I am growing towards the light. I feel the lightness of being at peace as I begin to accept myself completely.

Don't forget to use your prompts:
Today I will... Today I am... Today I think...
Today I feel... Today I believe... Today I trust... Today I can ...

EXERCISE:
I slow down and imagine unhooking myself from everything that is outside of me. I bring myself into my body and into the present moment. I am whole. I am here, right now, in this moment. I am at peace. I breathe in peace (breath). I breathe out everything that is not peace (breath). I breathe in peace (breath). I breathe out everything that is not peace (breath).

THURSDAY 1
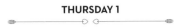

I bring my presence to the moment and I choose to be at peace.

FRIDAY 2
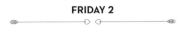

SATURDAY 3
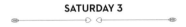

I feel safe to be with my difficult emotions.

SUNDAY 4
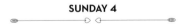

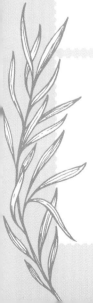

MONDAY 5
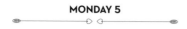

I connect to the energy of kindness and I am kind to myself.

TUESDAY 6
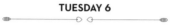

WEDNESDAY 7
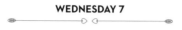

I feel my emotions and let them pass through me; they are not me.

THURSDAY 8
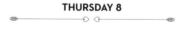

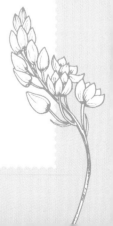

I walk away from drama and choose peace instead.

FRIDAY 9

SATURDAY 10

My day begins with peace and ends with peace.

SUNDAY 11

MONDAY 12

I allow myself to feel more at peace with myself.

TUESDAY 13

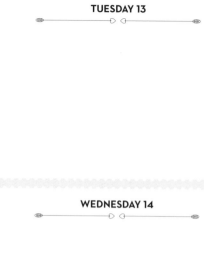

WEDNESDAY 14

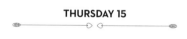

When I feel peace in my heart I see peace in the world.

THURSDAY 15

I experience the world through loving eyes.

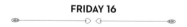

FRIDAY 16

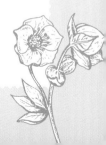

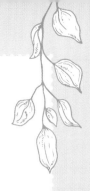

SATURDAY 17

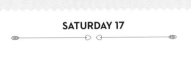

I release anything in me that is not at peace.

SUNDAY 18

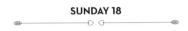

I slow down and bring myself back to the present moment.

MONDAY 19

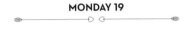

TUESDAY 20

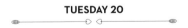

I feel safe to relax my mind and my body.

WEDNESDAY 21

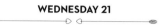

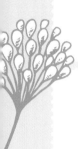

I am learning how to be completely at peace with myself.

THURSDAY 22

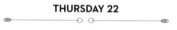

I am not afraid to ask for help.

FRIDAY 23

I let go of my need to cause myself emotional pain.

SATURDAY 24

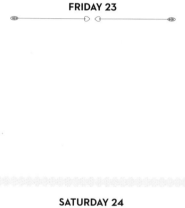

I let go of my need to cause myself emotional pain.

SUNDAY 25

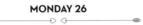

I am becoming my own best friend.

MONDAY 26

TUESDAY 27

I treat myself well and can look after myself.

WEDNESDAY 28

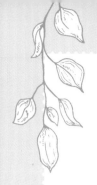

THURSDAY 29

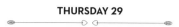

I am calm, I am safe, I am here, I am at peace.

FRIDAY 30

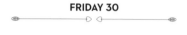

SATURDAY 31

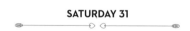

I send the energy of peace out into the world.

NOTES ON PEACE

March

WHAT DID I HAVE THE MOST DIFFICULTY WITH THIS MONTH?

HOW CAN I LOOK AFTER MYSELF NEXT MONTH?

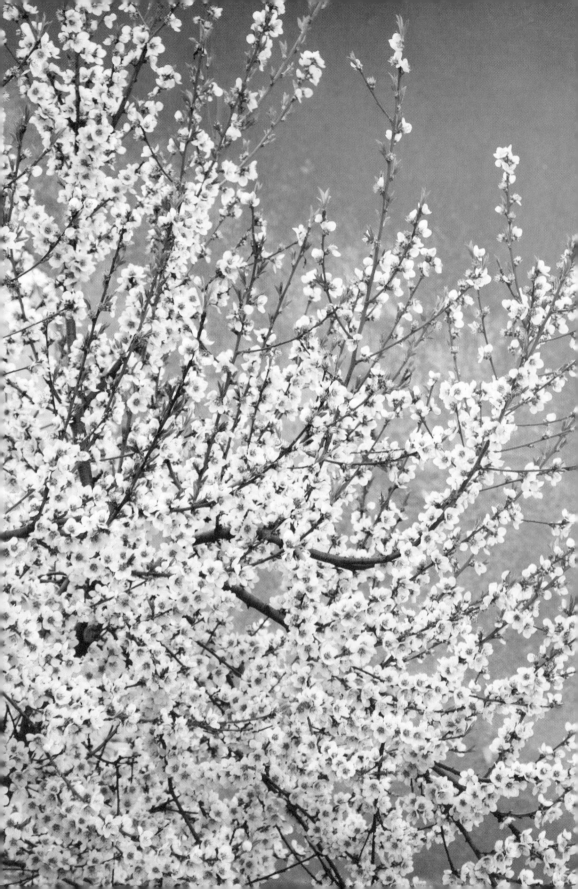

APRIL

PURIFICATION

This month I am ready for the next stage of my healing process.

'One of the most courageous decisions you'll ever make is to finally let go of what is hurting your heart and soul.'

Brigitte Nicole

APRIL

In order to create the space for more joy and love, I will
gently let go of heavy feelings like grief, anger, shame,
guilt and jealousy. I may also be carrying emotional
pain for my family and friends. When I take on other
people's emotional pain, they don't complete the
lessons they need to learn. I want to learn to not take
on others' pain and to set strong boundaries made of
compassion and love. I am not afraid to ask for help
or to share what I'm feeling with someone I trust. I am
ready and I feel safe enough to grow. I know that I am
looked after and that everything is as it should be.

Don't forget to use your prompts:
Today I will... Today I am... Today I think...
Today I feel... Today I believe... Today I trust... Today I can...

EXERCISE:
I imagine a fountain of love. I step into the fountain of love and it washes me clean.
I imagine that I am the mountain and my emotions are the weather.
The weather passes overhead and the mountain remains still.

SUNDAY 1

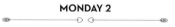

I accept myself just as I am.

MONDAY 2

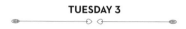

TUESDAY 3

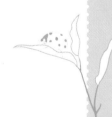

I give myself permission to let go of emotional pain.

WEDNESDAY 4

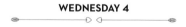

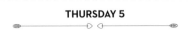

THURSDAY 5

I am patient and tolerant with myself.

FRIDAY 6

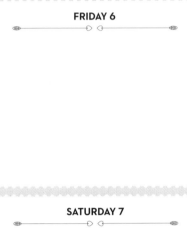

SATURDAY 7

I give myself and others the benefit of the doubt.

SUNDAY 8

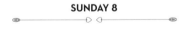

I am still learning and I am allowed to make mistakes.

MONDAY 9

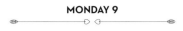

I breathe out anger, shame, guilt, frustration or jealousy.

TUESDAY 10

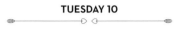

WEDNESDAY 11

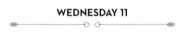

I fill myself with love so that I have love to give.

THURSDAY 12

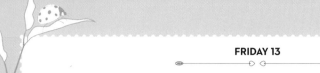

FRIDAY 13

SATURDAY 14

I am enough, just as I am.

SUNDAY 15

I give myself the time I need to make the changes I want to make.

MONDAY 16

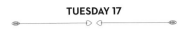

TUESDAY 17

I allow myself to feel emotions and then let them go.

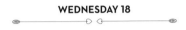

WEDNESDAY 18

I let go of my need to fix or change anything.

THURSDAY 19

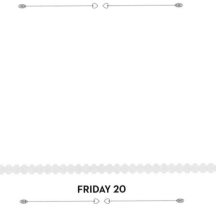

FRIDAY 20

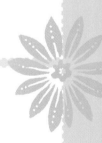

I pull myself out of the situation and back into me.

SATURDAY 21

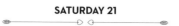

I slow down and choose peace in every situation.

SUNDAY 22

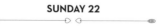

I don't need to compare myself to anyone else.

MONDAY 23

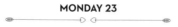

TUESDAY 24

It is safe for me to feel what I am feeling.

WEDNESDAY 25

I give myself permission to be happy.

THURSDAY 26

FRIDAY 27

Not everyone will like me and that's okay.

SATURDAY 28

SUNDAY 29

I allow myself to be completely who I am.

MONDAY 30

REVIEW YOUR POWER STATEMENT FOR THE YEAR

IS THERE ANYTHING YOU WISH TO CHANGE? REWRITE IT NOW, IN YOUR OWN WORDS.

April

HOW DO I FEEL AFTER ALL THE WORK THAT I HAVE DONE?

WHAT WOULD I LIKE TO INVITE INTO MY LIFE NOW?

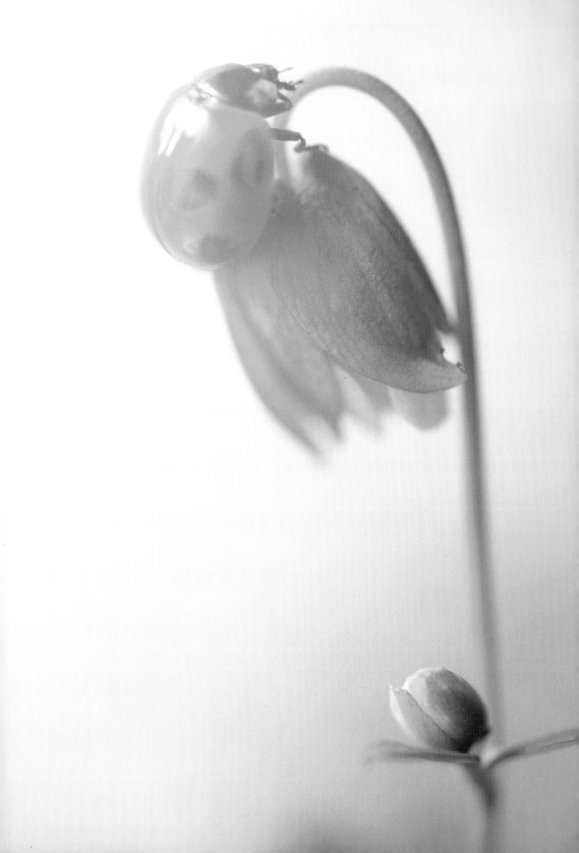

MAY

LOVE

This month I will immerse myself
in the energy of love.

'Your task is not to seek for love, but merely to seek
and find all the barriers within yourself that
you have built against it.'

Rumi

MAY

I am learning that true love is free from manipulation and control; love doesn't come with conditions. Conditions are created by people who are afraid they are not loveable just as they are. True love is an energy and there is enough for everyone. With the energy of love I can live a balanced life and truly accept who I am. I feel safe to let go of what blocks me from receiving love. It is safe to be open to love and to become a source of love.

Don't forget to use your prompts:
Today I will... Today I am... Today I think...
Today I feel... Today I believe... Today I trust... Today I can...

EXERCISE:
I imagine that I am a radio. I tune into the station of love. I breathe love in through the top of my head, I breathe in love all through my body. I feel the love flow down my arms and out of my hands and into everything I touch.

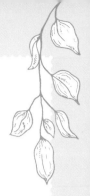

TUESDAY 1

I give permission for my heart to heal.

WEDNESDAY 2

THURSDAY 3

I slow down and feel the love around me.

FRIDAY 4

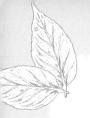

SATURDAY 5

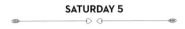

I am learning how to love myself more.

SUNDAY 6

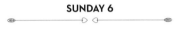

MONDAY 7

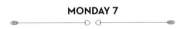

I accept myself just as I am in this moment.

TUESDAY 8

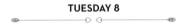

WEDNESDAY 9

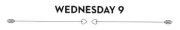

I give myself permission to receive love.

THURSDAY 10

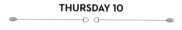

FRIDAY 11

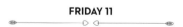

I let love into my heart and I expand.

SATURDAY 12

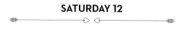

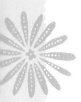

SUNDAY 13

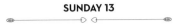

MONDAY 14

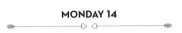

I am patient with others and see them through eyes of love.

TUESDAY 15

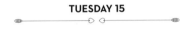

I can say no to things with love in my heart.

WEDNESDAY 16

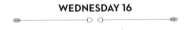

THURSDAY 17

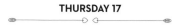

I open my heart to love and I shine my light in the world.

FRIDAY 18

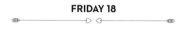

SATURDAY 19

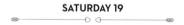

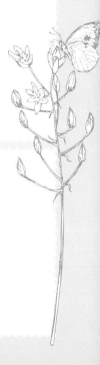

I deliberately choose love in every moment.

SUNDAY 20

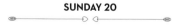

MONDAY 21

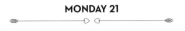

I connect my feet to the ground and feel safe to open my heart.

TUESDAY 22

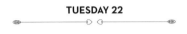

I bring myself back to a pure source of love.

WEDNESDAY 23

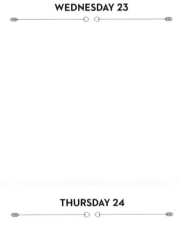

THURSDAY 24

Everyone deserves love and there is enough for everyone.

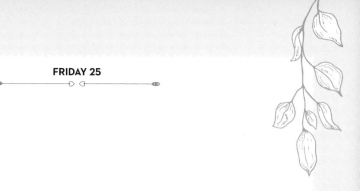

FRIDAY 25

Love flows through me. I am a conduit for love.

SATURDAY 26

SUNDAY 27

I do everything with love.

MONDAY 28

I draw energy from love and fill my environment with love.

May

WHAT CHANGED FOR ME WHEN I LET MORE LOVE INTO MY LIFE?

HOW CAN I BRING MORE LOVE INTO EVERYTHING THAT I DO?

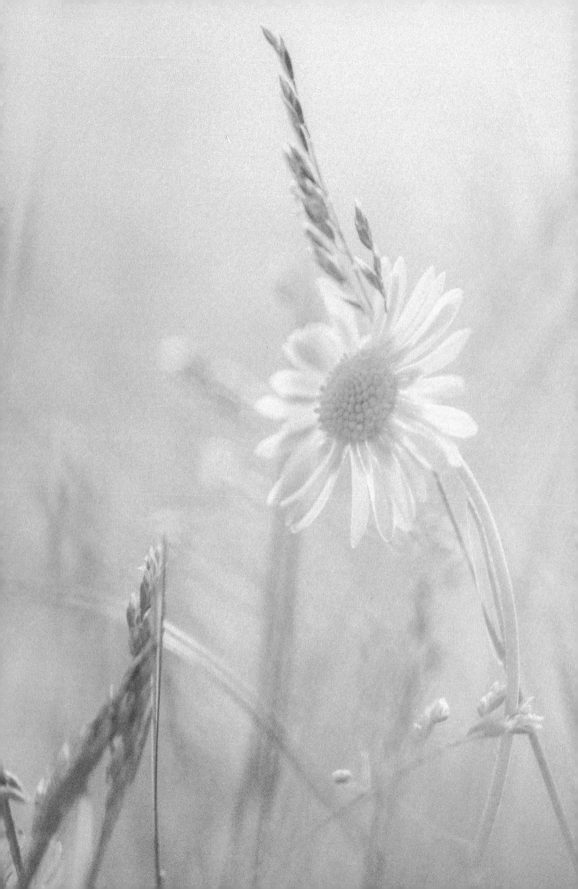

JUNE

BEAUTY

This month I open my eyes to discover
what beauty actually means to me.

'There are always flowers for those that want to see them.'

Henri Matisse

JUNE

When I allow myself to be the person that I truly am, I bring beauty into everything I do. Beauty and grace are wonderful energies that I can feel when I open my senses and give permission to receive. Material things can be beautiful, but I find more joy in grace, love, kindness and compassion. I release my fixed ideas of what is beautiful and allow life to surprise me with true beauty. I deliberately choose beauty and find that when I do this, more and more beauty comes into my life. I choose colours, smells and textures that are beautiful to me. I give myself permission to open my heart and let more beauty into my life.

Don't forget to use your prompts:
Today I will... Today I am... Today I think...
Today I feel... Today I believe... Today I trust... Today I can...

EXERCISE:
I bring myself into my heart centre. I open my heart to love. I let the energy of love flow right through my body. I let the energy of love flow into the ground and up to the sky. I see love, grace and beauty radiating everywhere.

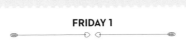

FRIDAY 1

I choose to resonate with the energy of beauty.

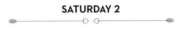

SATURDAY 2

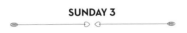

SUNDAY 3

I connect to the essence of beauty in all living things.

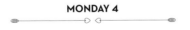

MONDAY 4

TUESDAY 5

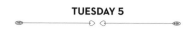

I feel safe and I am able to let go of guilt, shame, jealousy or fear.

WEDNESDAY 6

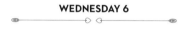

THURSDAY 7

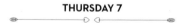

I find beauty in unexpected places.

FRIDAY 8

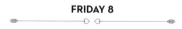

When I slow down and let love into my heart, I can see the beauty in the world.

SATURDAY 9

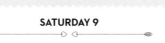

SUNDAY 10

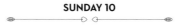

There is great beauty in small things.

MONDAY 11

I see what I see and I feel what I feel and I know that love exists.

TUESDAY 12

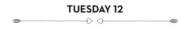

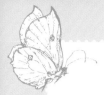

WEDNESDAY 13

THURSDAY 14

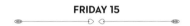

I choose to live a wholehearted life filled with compassion and love.

FRIDAY 15

I am beautiful like me and you are beautiful like you.

SATURDAY 16

SUNDAY 17

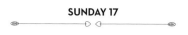

I know who I am and I treat myself well.

MONDAY 18

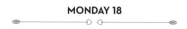

I let go of my need to control any situation.

TUESDAY 19

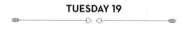

I choose kindness and compassion and I fill my life with beauty.

WEDNESDAY 20

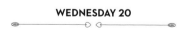

THURSDAY 21

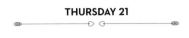

There can be beauty in difficult situations.

FRIDAY 22

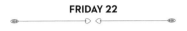

I trust in my intuition and I make good choices.

SATURDAY 23

SUNDAY 24

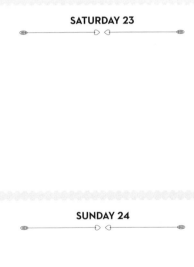

I slow down and take time to let beauty into my life.

MONDAY 25

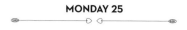

I look at the world with new eyes and a heart filled with love.

TUESDAY 26

WEDNESDAY 27

I open my heart to beauty and let more beauty into my world.

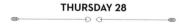

THURSDAY 28

I allow myself to feel all of my emotions and then let them go.

FRIDAY 29

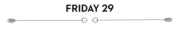

I am the centre of my universe; I bring myself into my centre.

SATURDAY 30

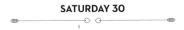

I open my heart and give myself the things I need.

NOTES ON BEAUTY

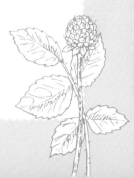

June

WHAT DOES BEAUTY MEAN TO ME?

HOW CAN I ADD MORE BEAUTY TO MY LIFE?

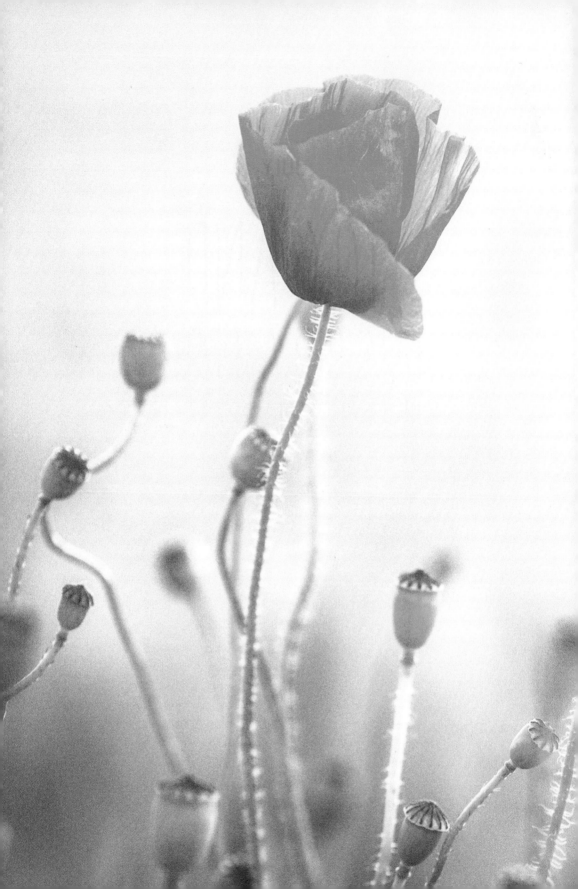

JOY AND INSPIRATION

This month I will explore how creative
I can be when my heart is filled with love.

'Joy comes to us in ordinary moments. We risk missing out
when we get too busy chasing the extraordinary.'

Brené Brown

JULY

I see the progress that I have made so far this year and I am filled
with joy. I resolve to express myself more and become more creative.
I know I don't have to make a career out of my talents but spending
time doing things that I love brings more joy into my world. I see time
in a different way as I live more in the present moment. I feel strongly
that I can invest more time in cultivating joy and being creative. I take
inspiration from the beauty in the nature that unfolds all around me.
I allow myself to have fun and to be lighter in my outlook on life. I
feel the ground beneath my feet and I let go of my need to carry
emotional pain. I am nicer to myself and I am nicer to be around too.
I notice that my relationships are improving. The more joy that I feel,
the less drama and conflict there is in my life.

Don't forget to use your prompts:
Today I will... Today I am... Today I think...
Today I feel... Today I believe... Today I trust... Today I can...

EXERCISE:
I imagine and write down what my life would be like if I had a never-ending supply of
money. What would I be doing? Where would I be going? What would I be seeing?
What would I look like? Who would be in my life? I consider that much of this can be
achieved without money. How can I capture the energy of this joyful and inspired
way of living, and bring it into my life right now?

SUNDAY 1

I allow joy into my life and I open my heart to joy.

MONDAY 2

TUESDAY 3

I trust my inner wisdom and give myself the things I need.

WEDNESDAY 4

THURSDAY 5

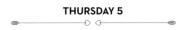

I recognise and allow my inner talent to shine through.

FRIDAY 6

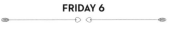

SATURDAY 7

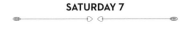

I feel safe to experiment and make mistakes.

SUNDAY 8

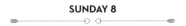

I allow myself the freedom to express myself in the world.

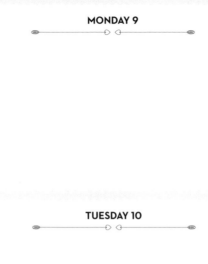

MONDAY 9

TUESDAY 10

I can spend time doing things that I love without guilt.

WEDNESDAY 11

THURSDAY 12

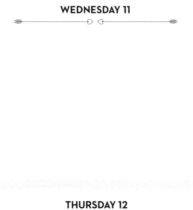

Life is more fun when I take the pressure off myself.

FRIDAY 13

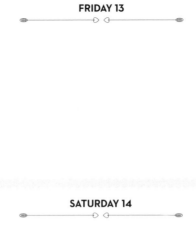

SATURDAY 14

I treat myself well and I know how to look after myself.

SUNDAY 15

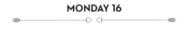

I deliberately choose things that make me happy.

MONDAY 16

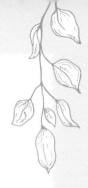

TUESDAY 17

I don't need to prove anything to anyone, not even myself.

WEDNESDAY 18

What is created in joy resonates with joy and amplifies joy.

THURSDAY 19

FRIDAY 20

I let go of my expectations and let love into my heart.

SATURDAY 21

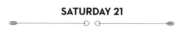

I give myself permission to express my creativity.

SUNDAY 22

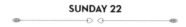

I will let my heart lead me today.

MONDAY 23

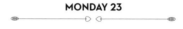

TUESDAY 24

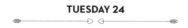

I create out of joy and love.

WEDNESDAY 25

I make space for inspiration and creativity.

THURSDAY 26

FRIDAY 27

I don't need to have all the answers today.

SATURDAY 28

I am grateful for all the joy in my life.

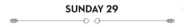

SUNDAY 29

I am learning how to create a life that I love.

MONDAY 30

TUESDAY 31

I feel the joy and freedom that comes from knowing who I am.

NOTES ON JOY AND INSPIRATION

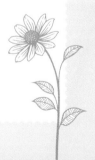

July

WHAT INSPIRED ME THE MOST THIS MONTH?

WHAT DOES JOY NOW MEAN TO ME?

AUGUST

COMPASSION

This month I notice how much easier it is for me to be kind to myself.

'Compassion for others begins
with kindness to ourselves.'

Pema Chodron

AUGUST

Compassion doesn't need to fix or change anything. Compassion and kindness are interlinked. When I am at peace my heart is wide open and filled with love, and compassion for myself and others flows in. I am becoming my own best friend. I am enjoying life more as I continue on this path. I know that in order for me to be compassionate I must slow down and be patient with myself and others. I give myself the space to do whatever it is that I need to do, so I can be more present in the moment. Compassion is becoming a way of being.

Don't forget to use your prompts:
Today I will... Today I am... Today I think...
Today I feel... Today I believe... Today I trust... Today I can...

EXERCISE:
I imagine unhooking myself from all the worries I carry, my own and others'. As I relax, I see my energy growing bigger and brighter. As I breathe and slow down I visualise strong boundaries appearing around me. I grow and expand until I feel better. I am confident in my personal space when I have more space to breathe.

WEDNESDAY 1

I open my heart to love and compassion.

THURSDAY 2

FRIDAY 3

I am compassionate with myself and others.

SATURDAY 4

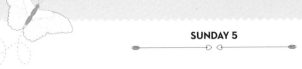

SUNDAY 5

I do not need to fix or change anyone else.

MONDAY 6

TUESDAY 7

I let go of the pressure I put on myself.

WEDNESDAY 8

I allow love, peace and kindness to surround me at all times.

THURSDAY 9

FRIDAY 10

I am doing the best that I can with what I know in this moment.

SATURDAY 11

SUNDAY 12

I slow down my thoughts and remember who I am.

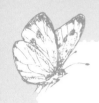

MONDAY 13
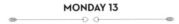

TUESDAY 14

I am able to give myself the love that I need.

WEDNESDAY 15

I feel safe to relax and be in the present moment.

THURSDAY 16

FRIDAY 17

I give myself the time that I need to do the things I need to do.

SATURDAY 18

I trust that everything is happening for a reason.

SUNDAY 19

MONDAY 20

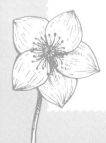

I don't need to have all of the answers.

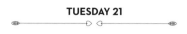

TUESDAY 21

I listen to my body and give it what it needs.

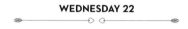

WEDNESDAY 22

Others are doing the best that they can with what they know in this moment.

THURSDAY 23

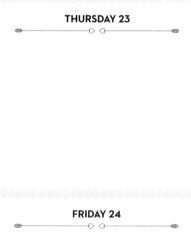

FRIDAY 24

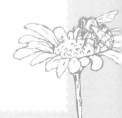

I bring myself back to my heart and connect to a source of love.

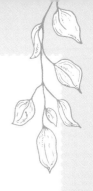

SATURDAY 25
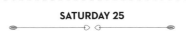

Love flows through me and around me.

SUNDAY 26
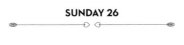

MONDAY 27
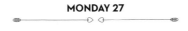

I breathe out heaviness and make more space within.

TUESDAY 28
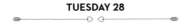

I can feel difficult emotions and let them go.

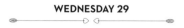

WEDNESDAY 29

I disconnect from fear and anger and I choose kindness and love.

THURSDAY 30

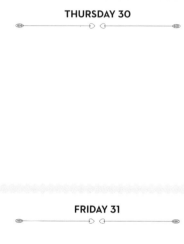

FRIDAY 31

My true source of happiness comes from within me.

NOTES ON COMPASSION

August

WHAT CHANGES IN THE MOMENT WHEN I REMEMBER TO CONNECT TO COMPASSION?

HOW CAN I BE EVEN MORE COMPASSIONATE TOWARDS MYSELF?

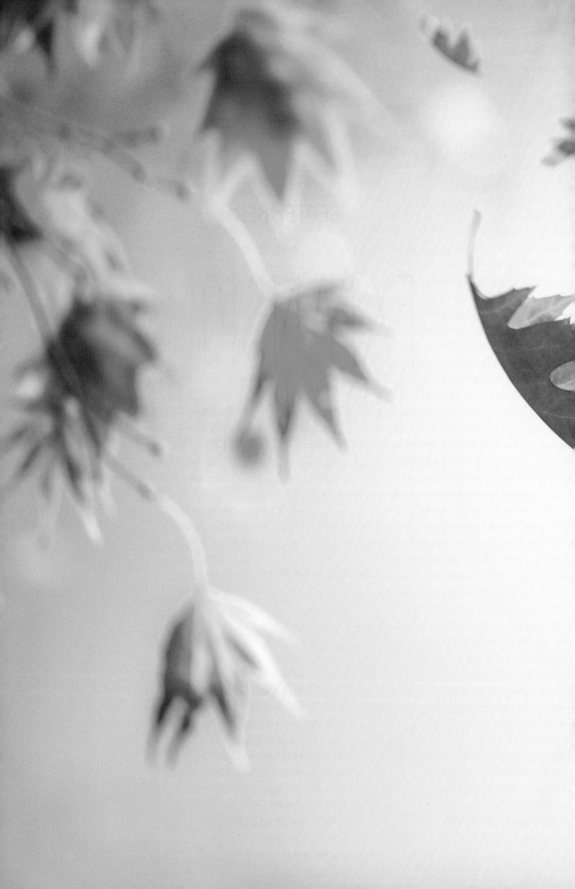

SEPTEMBER

EXPANSION AND GROWTH

This month I will continue my journey of healing and transformation.

'The one who would be constant in happiness must frequently change.'

Confucius

SEPTEMBER

I recognize that I have changed and grown. These changes may no longer resonate with the things that I have taken for granted in the past. I allow life to show me what else is weighing me down so that I can take the steps required to release it. I call on grace and beauty and the power of true love to give me the strength I need to let go of more emotional pain. I am willing to grow and expand and take up more space in the world. I allow myself to flourish and shine. I say yes to life.

Don't forget to use your prompts:
Today I will... Today I am... Today I think...
Today I feel... Today I believe... Today I trust... Today I can...

EXERCISE:
I slow down and bring my awareness into the present moment. I recognise how much I've grown. I visualise a bigger version of myself occupying more space in the world and I enlarge my self-conception accordingly. When I am grounded and my energy is expanded, my energy, confidence and self-worth increase and I can say yes to life!

SATURDAY 1

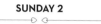

I am able to look after myself.

SUNDAY 2

MONDAY 3

I allow myself to be fully present in the world.

TUESDAY 4

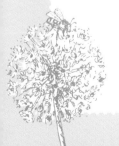

WEDNESDAY 5

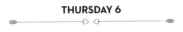

I surround myself with people and things that fill me with love.

THURSDAY 6

I am loving and kind to myself and others.

FRIDAY 7

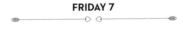

SATURDAY 8

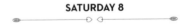

I release all judgement and see the world through compassionate eyes.

SUNDAY 9

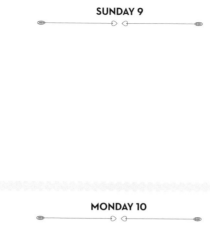

MONDAY 10

I can let go of things that I wasn't able to let go of before.

TUESDAY 11

I am safe, I am strong, I am here.

WEDNESDAY 12

THURSDAY 13

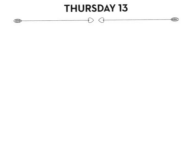

FRIDAY 14

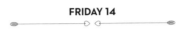

It is safe for me to say the things I need to say.

SATURDAY 15

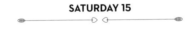

I am able to live a life filled with love.

SUNDAY 16

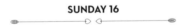

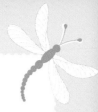

MONDAY 17

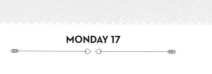

I enjoy life and the lessons that it brings me.

TUESDAY 18

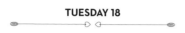

I am able to laugh at myself and not take things personally.

WEDNESDAY 19

I am allowed to make mistakes and grow from them.

FRIDAY 21

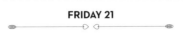

I no longer need to fix or change anything.

SATURDAY 22

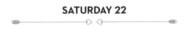

I can give myself all the things that I need.

SUNDAY 23

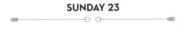

I have a wellspring of love within me.

MONDAY 24

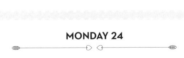

I have a wellspring of love within me.

TUESDAY 25

I am beginning to believe that anything is possible.

WEDNESDAY 26

THURSDAY 27

I am connected to beauty, joy and love.

FRIDAY 28

I bring love into everything I do.

SATURDAY 29

I give myself all the time I need to grow and heal.

SUNDAY 30

I allow the colours and magic of life to unfold.

REVIEW YOUR POWER STATEMENT FOR THE YEAR

REWRITE YOUR POWER STATEMENT SO IT IS IN ALIGNMENT WITH WHO YOU ARE NOW.

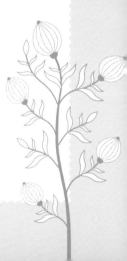

September

WHAT HAVE I BEEN ABLE TO LET GO OF THIS MONTH?

WHAT WOULD I LIKE TO INVITE INTO MY LIFE NEXT MONTH?

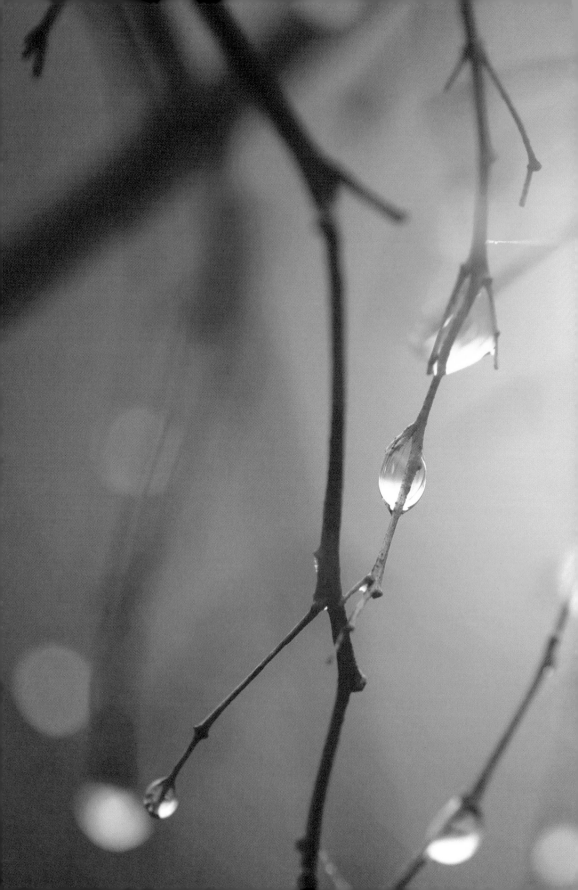

OCTOBER

HAPPINESS

**This month I will feel a freedom that
I have never experienced before.**

'I think everybody should get rich and famous
and do everything they ever dreamed of
so they can see that it's not the answer.'

Jim Carrey

OCTOBER

I am confident in who I am. I am spending more time doing things that I love. I don't get as upset as I used to by life's difficult situations. I find myself singing and smiling more often. I deliberately fill my days with beauty and love. I allow myself to try new things, to learn new skills and to bring more happiness into my life. I no longer depend on someone else to make me happy. I have found a source of internal happiness. I slow down and experience life in the present moment. I begin to imagine all the possibilities of my life. I constantly move in the direction of happiness. I realise that when I am happy I spread happiness wherever I go.

Don't forget to use your prompts:
Today I will... Today I am... Today I think...
Today I feel... Today I believe... Today I trust... Today I can...

EXERCISE:
I close my eyes and I become a bright shining light of happiness and joy. I feel my energy growing and filling the room. I grow and fill the building. I fill the street. I fill the town, the county and the country. I fill the world with this bright light of happiness, gratitude and love. I am here. I am here. I am here.

MONDAY 1

I feel the happiness that is within me.

TUESDAY 2

WEDNESDAY 3

I shine my light and fill the world with love and joy.

THURSDAY 4

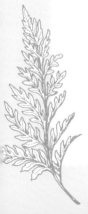

FRIDAY 5

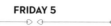

I feel safe to be in the world.

SATURDAY 6

SUNDAY 7

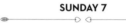

I allow myself to show up for life.

MONDAY 8

I spend more time doing the things I love.

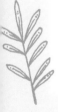

TUESDAY 9

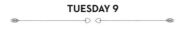

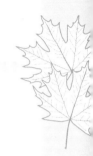

WEDNESDAY 10

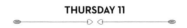

I relax and bring my awareness into the present moment.

THURSDAY 11

FRIDAY 12

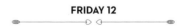

I give my body what it needs to radiate vibrant health.

SATURDAY 13

SUNDAY 14

I listen to my intuition and take action where needed.

MONDAY 15

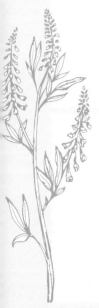

I breathe deeply, open my heart and drink from the beauty of life.

TUESDAY 16

WEDNESDAY 17

I can give myself anything I want.

THURSDAY 18

I listen to my inner wisdom and do what I need to do.

FRIDAY 19

SATURDAY 20

I choose to create my life from a place of love.

SUNDAY 21

I completely accept myself as I am.

MONDAY 22

I let go of anything that gets in the way of my happy life.

TUESDAY 23

WEDNESDAY 24

I am not afraid to make mistakes.

THURSDAY 25

When I connect to my inner light I can get through any situation.

FRIDAY 26

SATURDAY 27

I love learning new things and engaging with life.

SUNDAY 28

I release myself from my expectations of myself.

MONDAY 29

I am free to be who I am.

TUESDAY 30

I like who I am becoming.

WEDNESDAY 31

I am excited and inspired by the possibilities for my life.

NOTES ON HAPPINESS

REFLECTIONS ON

October

WHAT ARE THE KEY THINGS THAT I HAVE LEARNED ABOUT BEING HAPPY?

HOW CAN I KEEP CONNECTED TO MY INNER SOURCE OF HAPPINESS?

NOVEMBER

TRUST AND FAITH

This month I have a deeper
sense of who I am.

'Anything you can't control is for teaching
you how to let go and trust the Universe.'

Jackson Kiddard

NOVEMBER

I have moved from a state of not knowing who I am to a state of knowing. I have let go of the barriers to love and I now allow myself step into a life filled with joy, happiness and inspiration. When I accept who I am, I can accept others more fully for who they are, and give them the benefit of the doubt. I know that they are doing the best that they can with what they know right now. As I realise that I can make myself happy. I release everyone in my life from my expectations. I can see them and love them as they really are and not as I think they should be. I am more and more present in every moment of every day. I appreciate my life more fully. As time passes I no longer regret the things that I did or didn't do. Instead, I allow myself to experience what is here in front of me, right now.

Don't forget to use your prompts:
Today I will... Today I am... Today I think...
Today I feel... Today I believe... Today I trust... Today I can...

EXERCISE:
I think about something that I did or didn't do in the past and that I still regret. In my mind's eye, I see myself in that moment of time and space. I say, 'I know you did the best you could. I know more now and I may not do that now. However, I open my heart to kindness and compassion and I give you the benefit of the doubt. I forgive you completely. You are free.'

THURSDAY 1

I trust myself to make good choices.

FRIDAY 2

SATURDAY 3

I disconnect from my thoughts and I connect to the earth.

SUNDAY 4

MONDAY 5

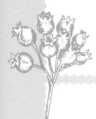

I know that I'm doing the best I can.

TUESDAY 6

WEDNESDAY 7

I forgive myself for things in the past.

THURSDAY 8

I am learning how to forgive others and let go of anger and pain.

FRIDAY 9

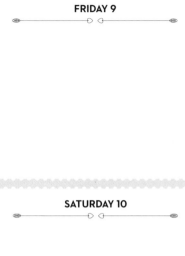

SATURDAY 10

Every day my light shines a little bit brighter.

SUNDAY 11

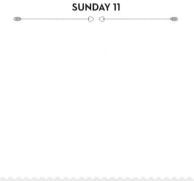

MONDAY 12

I know that I will meet the people I'm supposed to meet.

TUESDAY 13

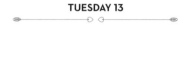

WEDNESDAY 14

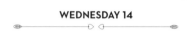

When my heart, mind and intuition are in agreement, good things always happen.

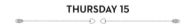

THURSDAY 15

I let go of my need to control the situation.

FRIDAY 16

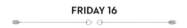

SATURDAY 17

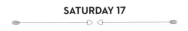

I feel safe to say the words I long to say.

SUNDAY 18

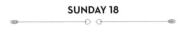

I disconnect from everything outside of me and reconnect to myself.

MONDAY 19

When I let love and happiness into my heart, it is reflected back on my life.

TUESDAY 20

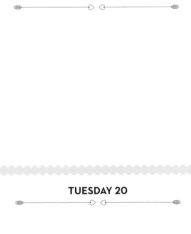

WEDNESDAY 21

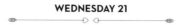

I breathe in peace and I breathe out all that is not peace.

THURSDAY 22

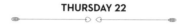

I make time to do the things that are truly important to me.

FRIDAY 23

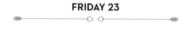

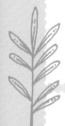

SATURDAY 24

I stop struggling with my expectations and let go of my resistance to life.

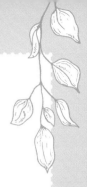

SUNDAY 25
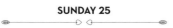

I hand my troubles over to the Universe.

MONDAY 26
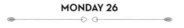

TUESDAY 27
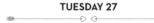

I fill my soul with love.

WEDNESDAY 28
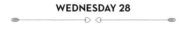

I trust my intuition and I take action when needed.

THURSDAY 29

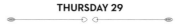

I step into the flow of life and let life carry me where it will.

FRIDAY 30

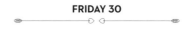

I trust that I can give myself everything I need.

WHAT I WOULD LIKE THE UNIVERSE TO TAKE CARE OF FOR ME:

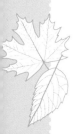

November

WHEN I CAN TRULY TRUST THAT ALL IS AS IT SHOULD BE, WHAT IS DIFFERENT FOR ME?

WHAT WORK DO I NEED TO DO TO CREATE A STRONGER SENSE OF TRUST AND FAITH?

TRUST AND FAITH

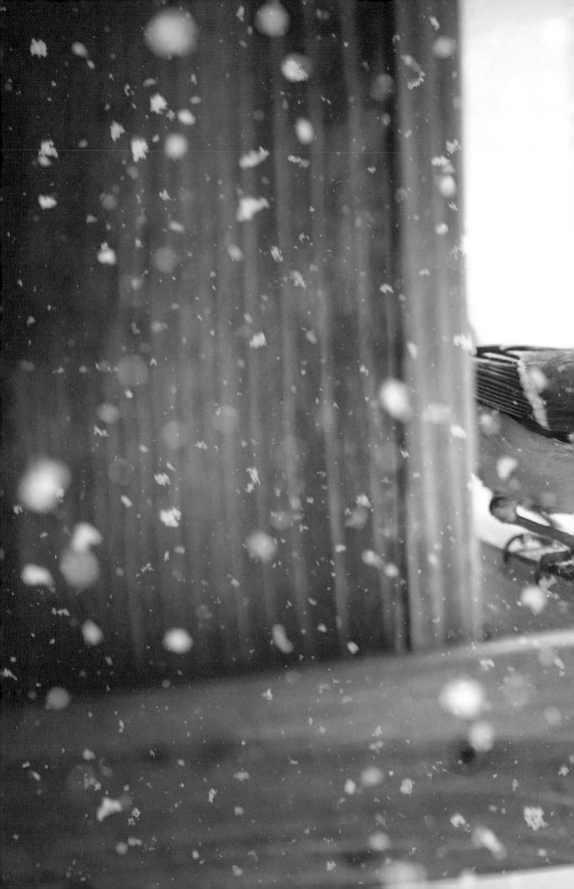

DECEMBER

GRATITUDE

This is the last month of the year.
I am so grateful for the work that I did
and now I feel all the benefits of it.

'Enjoy the little things, for one day
you may look back and realize they
were the big things.'

Robert Brault

DECEMBER

I know who I am and I recognise my talents. I allow myself to express myself. I am more tolerant and more patient with others. I have released people from my expectations. I can make myself happy. I have more beauty and love in my life. I look forward to next year and what it may bring. I use my imagination and my creativity to bring it into being. I will spend this month being grateful for all that I have experienced and all that is yet to come. I now understand that I am here on this planet to know who I am and to live a wholehearted life.

Don't forget to use your prompts:

Today I will... Today I am... Today I think...
Today I feel... Today I believe... Today I trust... Today I can...

EXERCISE:
I connect into gratitude and allow gratitude to flow through my body. I feel it flowing through my head, into my heart, down to my stomach, down my legs and into the ground. I breathe in gratitude and I breathe out anything that is not gratitude.
I am grateful for this day, for this life.

SATURDAY 1

I am grateful for the lessons that I have learned and the lessons I have yet to learn.

SUNDAY 2

MONDAY 3

I am grateful for all of my relationships.

TUESDAY 4

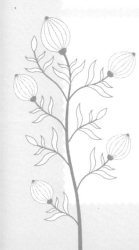

WEDNESDAY 5

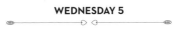

I slow down and appreciate what is right in front of me.

THURSDAY 6

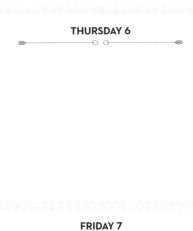

FRIDAY 7

I release my urgency and expectations and connect to a source of love.

SATURDAY 8

I am grateful that I no longer take things personally.

SUNDAY 9

MONDAY 10

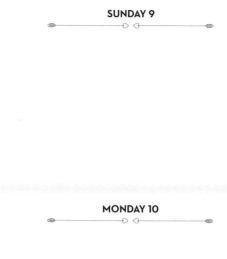

I fill my life with love and I am grateful for all that I have.

TUESDAY 11

WEDNESDAY 12

I am grateful for my body and all the work that it does for me.

THURSDAY 13

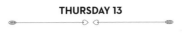

FRIDAY 14

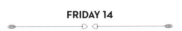

I open my heart and receive the love that is here for me.

SATURDAY 15

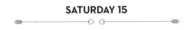

I am grateful for the food that I eat and the hands that prepare it.

SUNDAY 16

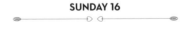

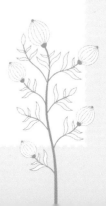

MONDAY 17

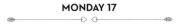

I embrace opportunities and experience life to the full.

TUESDAY 18

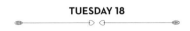

I am grateful for my voice and that I can say what I need to say.

WEDNESDAY 19

I trust that the Universe is looking after me in perfect ways.

THURSDAY 20

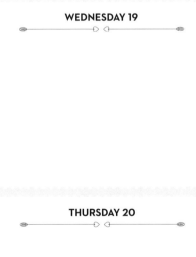

FRIDAY 21

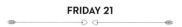

I am grateful for the things that I have in my life and the things that are yet to come.

SATURDAY 22

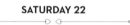

I open my heart to love and I let love into my life.

SUNDAY 23

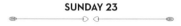

MONDAY 24

I am grateful for the beauty that surrounds me.

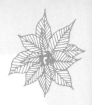

TUESDAY 25

I accept myself completely for who I am.

WEDNESDAY 26
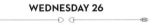

THURSDAY 27

I am grateful to be in the flow of life.

FRIDAY 28

I respect all human beings no matter where they are on their journey.

SATURDAY 29

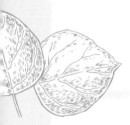

I respect myself and how far I have come.

SUNDAY 30

MONDAY 31

I am grateful that my life is filled with joy, hope and inspiration.

NOTES ON GRATITUDE

December

WHAT WAS MY BIGGEST LEARNING THIS MONTH?

HOW CAN I BRING GRATITUDE, LOVE, COMPASSION AND JOY INTO MY LIFE EVERY DAY?

REFLECTIONS ON

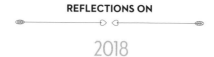

2018

THIS YEAR MY GREATEST LEARNING EXPERIENCE WAS...

MY MOST DIFFICULT MOMENT AND HOW I OVERCAME IT WAS...

REFLECTIONS ON

2018

MY PROUDEST ACHIEVEMENT THIS YEAR WAS...

NEXT YEAR I WOULD LIKE TO CREATE...

ACKNOWLEDGEMENTS

I want to say a huge thank you to Sarah Liddy, because without her vision and collaborative efforts this diary would never have come into being. Thank you to Jane Matthews who made my affirmations come alive with the most beautiful design, typography and layout. I also want to thank the team at Gill Books for all the enthusiasm and help in getting this book out there.

Gratitude and blessings to Marty Mulligan and Justin Moffat, the gatekeepers of the Hill of Usineach, for giving me permission to sit in stillness as long as I needed to receive inspiration from Lugh, Éiru and the land of Ireland.

And to you, dear reader – may you walk with grace and beauty, may your process of release be easy and profound, and may you step into your life of hope, joy and inspiration with love always in your heart.